Hummingbirth

A Sound Method for a Better Birth Experience

Ma Rae

Hummingbirth

This is a self published book written, edited, and designed by Ma Rae

First Edition
Copyright © 2024 **by** Ma Rae

ISBN number:
Printed in USA

Author's Note
No part of this publication may be reproduced, stored in a retrieval system, or transmitted in any form or by any means, electronic, mechanical, photocopying, recording, scanning, or otherwise, without the prior written permission of the author. This publication is designed to provide accurate and authoritative information in regards to the subject matter covered. It is sold with the understanding that neither the author nor the publisher is engaged in rendering legal, investment, accounting, or other professional services. While the author has used their best efforts in preparing this book, they make no representations or warranties with respect to the accuracy or completeness of the contents of this book and specifically disclaim any implied warranties of merchantability or fitness for a particular purpose. No warranty may be created or extended by sales representatives or written sales materials. The advice and strategies contained herein may not be suitable for your situation. You should consult with a professional when appropriate. The author shall not be liable for any loss of profit or any other commercial damages, including but not limited to special, incidental, consequential, personal, or other damages.

Table of Contents

Dedication

This book is dedicated to the mothers who came before
us—
keepers of sacred wisdom,
weavers of life's ancient song.

Your strength echoes in our hearts,
your courage hums through our bodies,
and your love lights the path to better births.

Through you, we remember,
we rise,
and we reclaim the power of our beginnings.

This is for you. This is because of you.

Introduction: Why Humming?

The Unexpected Power of Sound in Labor

Welcome! If you're here, you're likely on a quest to make the birthing process something more than a haze of discomfort, nerves, and medical jargon. Maybe you're hoping for a shortcut, a method to smooth out the bumps, or just a small tip that might help. The idea of humming might sound curious, or even absurd, but stay with me—I promise you, there's something to this.

As a midwife for over four decades, I've seen birthing techniques come and go. But humming is ancient and real, simple yet profound. It's natural, familiar, and powerful. The science behind it is fascinating, and the results I've witnessed firsthand are nothing short of inspiring. Humming helps to focus the mind, relax the body, and, yes, even speed things up.

But more than that, humming can help dissolve the fear that often shadows childbirth. There's something almost primal in it—a reminder of the ancient wisdom our bodies already carry. Humming, when done with intention, can become a form of strength, a way to turn inward and reclaim power over the birth process. I want this book to be your guide in doing just that, empowering you with a tool that's been in our DNA for as long as humans have been bringing new life into the world.

So, grab a cozy seat, and let's dive into a practice that can make your birthing journey not only more bearable but also profoundly fulfilling. You'll come away with a fresh approach to labor that taps into the very essence of who you are.

One

The Power of Humming in Birth – Where Ancient Wisdom Meets Modern Science

Welcome to the hum—the unassuming little sound that's going to be your new best friend during labor. You might be surprised at the idea of humming your way through contractions, but this humble technique holds a surprising power. Not only is it deeply grounding and easy to access, but it's also backed by some remarkable science. Humming has a profound effect on your body and mind during labor, engaging natural mechanisms that support pain relief, relaxation, and focus. In this chapter, we're going to unpack the "why" and "how" behind humming, from its impact on your hormones to its influence on your breathing.

The Physiological Benefits: Endorphins and Natural Pain Relief

Let's start with a little chemistry lesson. Humming, like other forms of vocalization, stimulates the release of endorphins—the body's natural pain relievers.[1] These feel-good chemicals work a lot like morphine, dulling pain while also lifting your mood. When labor intensifies, humming becomes more than just a comforting sound; it becomes an active tool in your body's fight against pain. By encouraging the flow of endorphins, you're setting yourself up to experience each contraction with a touch more ease and grace.

Imagine each hum as a little pulse of relief. With every vibration, endorphins flow, bringing you closer to a calm state of mind and body. This isn't just about feeling better; it's about transforming the way you experience pain. Instead of bracing yourself against it, you're moving with it, allowing each contraction to come and go like waves, with a steady hum helping you stay afloat.

Humming and the Vagus Nerve: Activating the Relaxation Response

Here's where the science gets fascinating. When you hum, you activate a remarkable part of your nervous system called the vagus nerve, a major player in the body's "rest and digest" response.(2) This nerve is like a built-in relaxation switch that helps lower your heart rate, reduce blood pressure, and bring you back to a state of calm. Humming is one of the most effective ways to stimulate the vagus nerve, which, in turn, helps reduce stress and anxiety, creating a peaceful environment for labor.

Think of your vagus nerve as your calm companion during birth, and the hum as the key that activates it. When you hum, you're signaling your body to relax, to breathe deeper, to slow down. This gentle activation creates a sense of safety and calm, helping you to stay present and grounded.

The Nitric Oxide Boost: Breath, Immunity, and Pain Modulation

One lesser-known benefit of humming is its role in boosting nitric oxide (NO) levels.(3) Studies, including one from the American Journal of Respiratory and Critical Care Medicine, show that humming can significantly increase nitric oxide in the nasal passages. This gas isn't just a random byproduct—it's a powerful ally during labor. Nitric oxide acts as a natural sterilizer, helping to cleanse the air you breathe. Additionally, it increases arterial oxygenation, which means more oxygen for both you and your baby.

Not only does nitric oxide enhance oxygen flow, but it also plays a role in pain modulation. Research has shown that NO can lower blood pressure and reduce pain perception. Each time you hum, you're not only calming yourself but actively supporting your body's ability to deliver oxygen more efficiently, making the entire birth process safer and more manageable.

Humming and Oxytocin: Strengthening the Bond, Supporting Contractions

Humming has a beautiful relationship with oxytocin, also known as the 'trust hormone' or "love hormone." This is the same hormone released during a loving touch, a warm hug, nursing a baby or, yes, labor. Oxytocin is crucial in childbirth, facilitating uterine contractions and enhancing the bond between mother and baby. When you hum, you release oxytocin, which not only supports the progress of labor but also brings a sense of connection and empowerment.(4)

Each hum is like a gentle reminder to yourself: you are doing this, you are strong, and you are in harmony with your body. This oxytocin-rich environment fosters a positive experience, one where labor feels less like something to "get through" and more like something to engage with, to ride with grace.

Breathing with Intention: How Humming Supports Rhythmic Breathing

One of the reasons humming works so well in labor is that it naturally supports rhythmic, controlled breathing. As you hum, you slow down your exhale, creating a deep, calming breathing pattern. This steady rhythm encourages relaxation by reducing stress hormones like cortisol, helping you stay focused and energized.(5)

With each hum, you're sending a message to your brain: "I am safe. I am calm." This approach to breathing helps conserve energy and provides a focal point that keeps you grounded.

Instead of getting swept up in the intensity of contractions, you're guiding your body into a pattern of rhythm and release, making labor feel less chaotic and more like a dance.

Humming as Pain Modulation: Rewiring the Brain's Response to Pain

There's also a fascinating neurological element to humming. Studies have shown that vocalization—including humming—can alter the brain's processing of pain signals. When you hum, you're essentially shifting the brain's attention away from the intensity of contractions, changing how it perceives pain.

By providing a focus on sound and vibration, humming creates a "distraction" for the brain, allowing you to stay more present and in control. Instead of solely concentrating on the pain, you're tuning into the soothing vibrations resonating within you, transforming the experience of labor into something more manageable. Each hum becomes an anchor, helping you to stay grounded and focused even as contractions build.

The Mental Benefits: Focus, Presence, and Inner Calm

In the midst of labor, the mind can easily wander—often to places of worry or self-doubt. Humming provides a point of focus, a way to redirect your attention and connect with the present moment. When you hum, you're not only creating sound; you're fostering a sense of inner calm and confidence, a reminder that you are in control, that you are capable.

This focus doesn't just help you manage pain; it brings you into a space of trust with your own body. Humming offers a moment-by-moment presence, allowing you to stay connected to each sensation, each contraction, without getting overwhelmed.

Enhancing Heart Rate Variability: Building Resilience in Labor

Finally, let's talk about heart rate variability (HRV), which is a key measure of how well you handle stress. Research has shown that humming can improve HRV, an indicator of resilience and recovery. When you hum, you're helping your body shift from "fight or flight" mode into a more relaxed state, one that's primed for the intensity of labor.

Each hum enhances your HRV and reduces blood pressure,(6) supporting your ability to adapt and respond calmly as labor progresses. You're giving yourself a tool not only to manage pain but to strengthen your body's natural resilience, preparing yourself to meet the challenges ahead with a steady heart and a steady breath.

A Sound of Ancient Wisdom

Humming isn't a new concept; it's an ancient practice, a sound that has accompanied countless births before yours. Women have been humming, chanting, and singing their way through labor for centuries, tapping into the wisdom of the body to ease pain and find rhythm. By embracing this sound, you're connecting with a lineage of mothers who trusted their instincts, who knew that there was power in simple, natural sounds. You're not just learning a technique—you're reclaiming an ancient wisdom, one that has always been a part of birth.

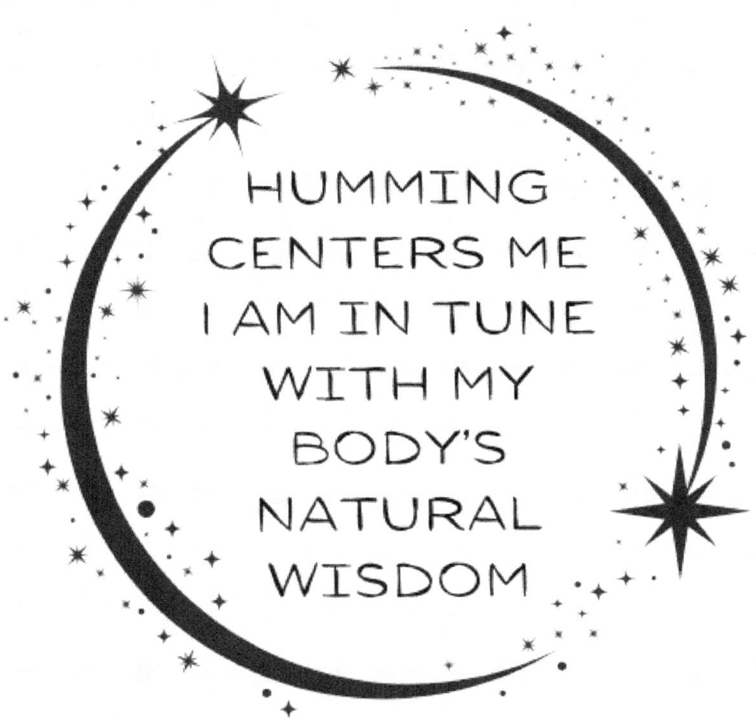

HUMMING
CENTERS ME
I AM IN TUNE
WITH MY
BODY'S
NATURAL
WISDOM

Two

The Labor Connection – Why Humming Works for Pain and Progression

Let's be honest: labor has a reputation. It's the marathon we all dread, the great ordeal whispered about with wide eyes at baby showers and among friends who've "been there." Pain, unpredictability, intensity—labor promises to deliver it all. But what if, instead of bracing ourselves to just endure it, we learned to work *with* it?

Enter humming. Think of it as an old friend, steady and true, a sound that's here to hold your hand and remind you that labor doesn't have to be a battle. It can be something you move through, a rhythm you find and stay with as each contraction comes and goes. Because here's the thing: labor isn't out to get you. It's trying to *work with you* to bring this baby into the world, and the hum? It's there to help you stay on that team.

Tuning In: Humming as a Way to Set the Stage for Birth

Now, here's where things get fascinating. When we think of pain relief, most of us picture numbing the area or "taking something for it." But humming doesn't numb or distract; it *redirects*. Think of it like steering a boat—you don't eliminate the waves, but you learn to ride them more skillfully. Each hum creates a soothing vibration that aligns with your body's rhythm, allowing you to feel the contraction without getting lost in it.

The low, continuous sound of a hum keeps your breath steady, your heart rate calm. It's a gentle yet powerful way of saying, "I'm here, I'm steady, and I've got this." And believe me, there's something incredibly empowering about discovering that, even in the most intense moments, you have that hum to ground you.

Hummingbirth

Pain Isn't the Villain, It's the Guide

I know it sounds a bit radical to suggest we don't view pain as the enemy. After all, our natural instinct is to push pain away, bury it, or mask it. But in birth, pain is actually part of the roadmap. It's telling us where we are, what's happening, and how we can help move things along.

That's where humming becomes even more powerful—it doesn't numb the sensation, but rather it transforms the relationship you have with it. A hum allows you to acknowledge the sensation, without getting swept away by it. Think of it as taking the volume knob on pain and dialing it back just a few notches.

The hum's vibration travels through the diaphragm and the belly, gently encouraging the uterus to contract more effectively. Every vibration strengthens your bond with your body, reminding you that you are *built for this*. You're not fighting against labor; you're leaning into it, riding each wave with a rhythm that has been within you all along.

Finding the Groove in the Groove

Let's get practical for a second. You may be wondering, "When do I start humming, and what's the magic rhythm?" Well, that's the beauty of it: there's no one-size-fits-all hum. The trick is finding *your* groove—your unique frequency and rhythm that feels natural, comforting, and, most importantly, *yours.*

A good place to start is with a low, gentle hum at the start of each contraction. You'll find that over time, the hum may start to take on a rhythm of its own, moving with your breath and the natural pattern of your contractions. And don't be surprised if you even start to hum without thinking about it. This is your body tapping into its own wisdom, doing what it knows best.

Imagine labor as a dance, where each hum becomes a step, each vibration a note in a song only you can hear. And as you sink deeper into that rhythm, you'll start to feel less like someone struggling against the waves and more like a woman moving with them, confident in her own power.

Embracing Your Own Soundtrack

Labor isn't about perfection or getting it "right"; it's about finding what works, what feels good, and what brings you that one small step closer to meeting your baby. Humming, for some, becomes a kind of soundtrack—something that brings focus, relieves fear, and helps them connect to a process as old as time. For others, it might be a soft reminder in the background, a quiet hum only heard now and then.

Whichever way humming works for you, let it be a source of strength. Let it be a reminder that, even in the rawest, realest moments, you have this incredible tool, this ancient, intuitive practice that's been with birthing women for centuries.

Because at the end of the day, that's the beauty of labor: it's yours. Every hum, every breath, every vibration is yours. So go ahead—trust the rhythm, embrace the sound, and let it carry you through. You are more than capable, and this hum? It's here to remind you every step of the way.

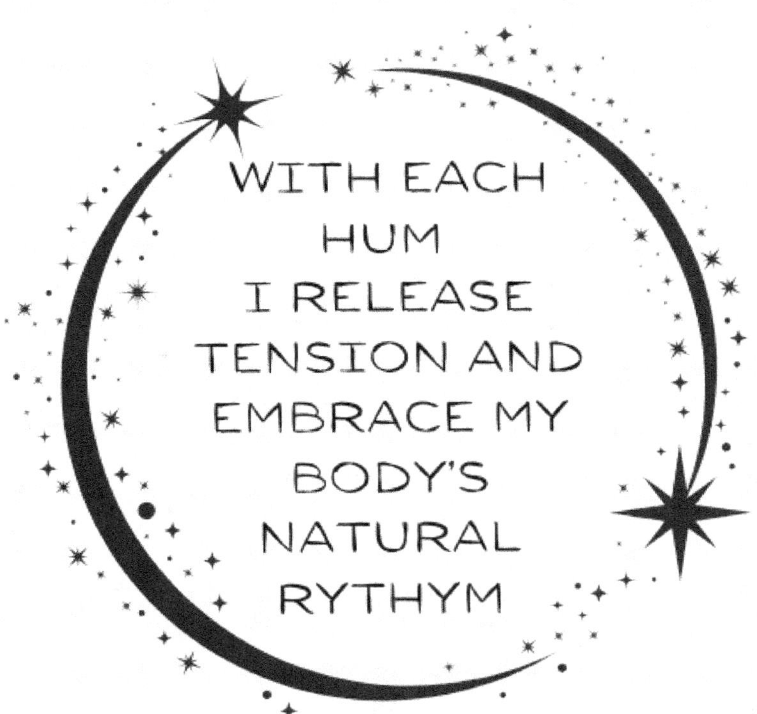

WITH EACH
HUM
I RELEASE
TENSION AND
EMBRACE MY
BODY'S
NATURAL
RYTHYM

Three

Getting Started with Humming – Techniques to Practice Before Labor

Let's get comfortable with our new friend, the hum, before the big day arrives. Because just like any skill, humming gets better—and feels more natural—with a bit of practice. Think of this chapter as a warm-up, a way to get acquainted with a sound that'll soon become one of the most valuable tools in your birthing toolkit.

The Gentle Art of Tuning In

So, where to begin? The good news is, you don't need fancy equipment or a quiet mountaintop retreat. Humming is simple, portable, and, best of all, it's already within you. But to make it work well for labor, we want to get familiar with how it feels, what it sounds like, and how it impacts your body. It's like learning to play an instrument—your own voice—and getting a sense of the rhythm and resonance that feels best to you.

Let's start with a few deep breaths. Inhale slowly, letting your belly expand, and then exhale with a gentle, steady hum. Nothing forced, nothing fancy—just a soft, continuous hum that rolls off your vocal cords and resonates in your chest. You might notice a slight vibration, a warmth that seems to spread from your core outward. That's what we're looking for, that grounding sensation that connects your breath, your voice, and your body.

Hummingbirth

Finding Your Frequency: High, Low, and In-Between

Now, here's the fun part. Not all hums are created equal! Each of us has a "sweet spot," a pitch that feels particularly calming, strong, or just *right*. Some women find that a low, deep hum feels most comforting, while others prefer a mid-range tone. There's no wrong way to hum—this is about finding your unique rhythm, the sound that feels most resonant and soothing for *you.*

Take a few moments to try humming at different pitches. Start low, then go a bit higher, and notice how each one feels. You'll start to get a sense of the sounds that feel grounding, the ones that seem to "click" with your breath and heartbeat. Remember, there's no rush; the hum you choose now doesn't have to be the hum you use in labor. This is about building familiarity and comfort with a sound that, soon enough, will feel as natural as breathing.

Practice, Pause, Repeat: Building a Humming Habit

Like any good tool, humming is most effective when it's been broken in a bit. Try working it into your daily routine—during a quiet moment in the morning, in the shower, or while winding down in the evening. You don't have to hum for long; even a few minutes a day can help your body "remember" the sound, making it easier to call upon when labor begins.

And here's the beauty of it: the more you practice, the more humming becomes second nature. You'll find yourself starting to hum almost automatically when you feel stressed, uncomfortable, or simply in need of a little grounding. That's the body's way of saying, "This works. Let's keep this handy."

Hummingbirth

Humming for Relaxation and Pain Relief

Even before labor, humming can help you connect with your body's natural relaxation response. Imagine this: you're feeling the usual aches and pains that can accompany pregnancy—the swollen feet, the backache that's been your constant companion for weeks now. Try taking a deep breath and releasing it with a hum, allowing the vibration to resonate down through your belly and into those sore muscles. It's a small thing, but you might find it brings just a bit of relief, a gentle reminder that your body has ways of easing itself.

Practice humming when you're feeling tense or achy, and notice how it shifts your awareness from the pain to the rhythm of the sound. Each hum is like a small retreat, a way of stepping back from discomfort and grounding yourself in something soothing and familiar. This is the same technique you'll be using during labor, just with a different kind of intensity.

Visualization and Humming: Bringing the Sound to Life

Once you're comfortable with the basics, it can be helpful to add a visualization exercise to your humming practice. Imagine each hum as a wave—one that rolls through your body, softening and relaxing every muscle it touches. Picture it spreading through your chest, down into your belly, easing any tension and carrying it away. This visualization can make your hum feel even more effective, helping you connect the sound to a sense of physical release.

In the same way, you might visualize your hum as a cocoon of sound surrounding you, a kind of shield that buffers you from anxiety and stress. With every hum, you're building a layer of calm that's uniquely yours—a sound that brings you back to yourself, even in the most intense moments.

Hummingbirth

At the end of this book, you'll find a link to a set of guided humming meditations created to support you through the ups, downs, and wild beauty of pregnancy and childbirth. I designed these meditations to help you find calm, ease discomfort, and connect more deeply with your body and baby. They're practical, grounding, and a reminder that you're stronger and more capable than you might feel in the moment. Let these meditations be steady companions on your journey to a more peaceful and empowered birth.

Preparing for the Big Day

Remember, this is your practice, your sound. There's no right or wrong way to approach it. Humming is like an old folk remedy passed down from generation to generation—intuitive, adaptable, something you make your own. The more you practice, the more you're not only preparing for labor; you're cultivating a sense of calm and confidence that will serve you long beyond birth.

As you move forward, know that each hum is helping you lay the groundwork for a birth that is deeply connected to your own rhythm, your own power. You're building muscle memory, yes, but also emotional memory—the knowledge that you have what it takes to meet labor with strength and calm.

So, go ahead, hum to your heart's content. Let it become part of your day, part of your journey to birth. Soon enough, you'll find that your body remembers the hum in every contraction, every breath, every moment that brings you closer to meeting your baby. And that, dear reader, is the quiet magic of the hum—a simple sound, yes, but one that carries the wisdom of centuries, resonating within you, ready to be called upon when it matters most.

Hummingbirth

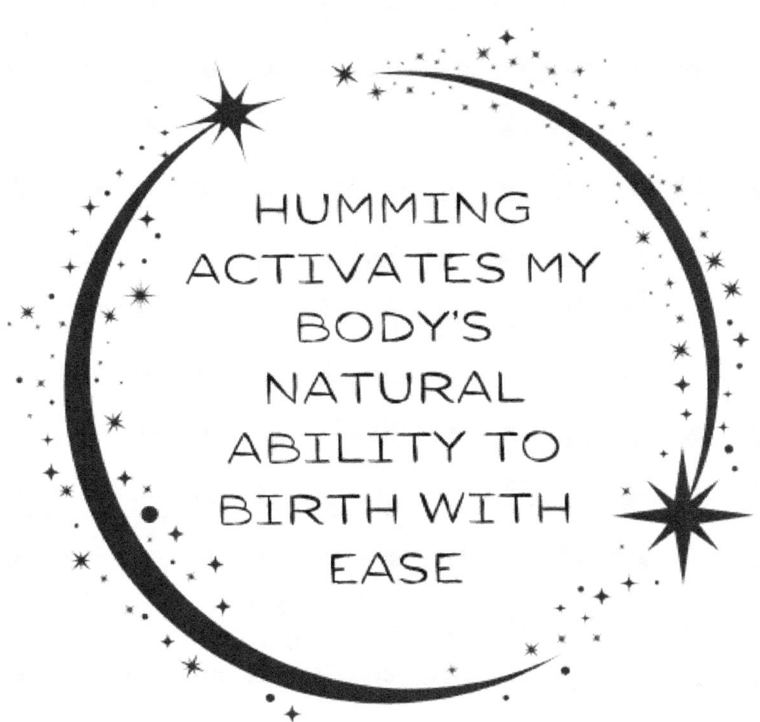

HUMMING
ACTIVATES MY
BODY'S
NATURAL
ABILITY TO
BIRTH WITH
EASE

Four

Early Labor – Finding Your Rhythm as the Waves Begin

So here you are. The bags are packed, the baby clothes are neatly folded, and now you're waiting for that first whisper, that quiet nudge from your body saying, "It's time." Early labor can feel like a mystery—a time of wondering, second-guessing, and, let's be real, a whole lot of clock-watching. Is this it? Am I ready? And maybe: What if I forgot everything?

But early labor is also your chance to settle into your groove, to get comfortable with the rhythm that will carry you through. This stage is all about listening, trusting, and yes, finding that steady hum. Because if labor is a song, early labor is the quiet intro, the place where you start to feel the beat before the chorus kicks in.

Humming as a Grounding Practice

As you begin to feel those first stirrings, those soft contractions coming and going like the tide, it can be tempting to get ahead of yourself—to think about the hours ahead, the intensity that might come. But here's where humming becomes a gift. It brings you right back to now, to this breath, to this moment.

In these early stages, your hum doesn't need to be powerful or intense. Instead, let it be soft and grounding, like the background music to a scene you're easing into. When you feel the first inklings of a contraction, take a slow, deep breath and release it with a gentle hum. Keep it quiet, calm. You're not pushing through anything just yet; you're simply getting acquainted with the rhythm your body is setting.

This early hum is like dipping your toe into the water before the waves really start rolling. Each hum can remind you that, yes, this is happening, and yes, you are absolutely ready. With each soft vibration, you're giving your body a gentle "I'm here. Let's do this."

Letting Go of "Performance"

One of the most beautiful things about humming is that it has no rules. You don't have to get it "right." Early labor can feel a bit like you're in a waiting room, wondering if you're doing everything you're supposed to be doing. But with humming, there's no checklist. There's only the sound, the sensation, and your own comfort.

So let go of the idea that this stage has to look any certain way. You're not auditioning for labor; you're easing into it. Every woman's labor is different, and every labor has its own unique rhythm. Let the hum become a companion, not a chore, a way of connecting with what feels right to you in the moment.

Embracing the Small Breaks

Early labor contractions are usually manageable, with long, luxurious breaks in between. These breaks are your body's way of saying, "Pace yourself." It's in these moments that the hum can be a balm, a way to fill the space and keep yourself centered without getting lost in anticipation.

During these breaks, keep your hum soft and relaxed. Think of it as a way of settling in, making yourself comfortable. It doesn't need to be loud or forceful—just steady. Like sitting down in a favorite chair, the hum is a way of saying, "I'm here, I'm present, and I'm okay."

And if there's one thing I want you to remember in this stage, it's this: You have time. This isn't a race; it's a process. The hum is a gentle reminder that you can take each contraction as it comes, one by one, moment by moment.

Moving with Your Hum

For some women, early labor is a time of rest, of leaning into stillness. For others, it's a time of movement, of pacing, of finding ways to stay active and release a bit of that nervous energy. Wherever you fall on the spectrum, know that there's no wrong way to be here.

If you're feeling restless, try moving with your hum. Walk around the room, sway your hips, or take slow, grounding steps as you breathe in, hum out. Let the hum become part of your movement, an anchor that keeps you connected to your breath and body. With each step, each hum, you're saying yes to the process, letting it unfold naturally and in its own time.

And if you're more inclined to settle in and rest, let the hum be your heartbeat. Keep it low, keep it steady. Whether you're lying down or nestled in a cozy chair, allow the vibration to remind you that labor is a marathon, not a sprint. These early moments are a warm-up, a gentle way to ease yourself into the journey.

Staying Present, Staying Calm

Early labor has a way of inviting thoughts to drift. You may find yourself thinking about what's coming next, worrying about how you'll handle the intensity, or wondering if you're doing enough. But here's the beauty of the hum: it keeps you present. It brings you back from that mental wandering, back into your body, back into the moment.

Each hum is a way to remind yourself that you are here, now, and that is enough. You don't need to solve or anticipate the rest of labor just yet. You only need to meet this moment, this breath, and let the hum be your guide. The contractions will come and go, like waves, and with each one, you'll find a little more strength, a little more confidence in the rhythm that's taking shape.

Preparing for What's Ahead, One Hum at a Time

As you move through early labor, remember that each hum is a building block. You're creating a foundation, laying down layer upon layer of calm, confidence, and connection. This is your time to practice, to find your rhythm, to get comfortable with the sound and sensation of the hum. You're setting the stage for the rest of the journey, allowing yourself to become more familiar with this simple yet powerful tool.

And if early labor takes a while, that's okay. Every contraction, every hum is bringing you one step closer. Let this stage be a time of patience, of gentle acceptance, of embracing the slow, natural rhythm of birth. You are exactly where you need to be, moving forward with each breath, each sound, each heartbeat.

So, take your time. Sink into the hum, let it become a part of you, and trust that this is just the beginning of a journey you are beautifully equipped to navigate. Early labor is your time to settle in, to find your groove, to discover the power that's been within you all along.

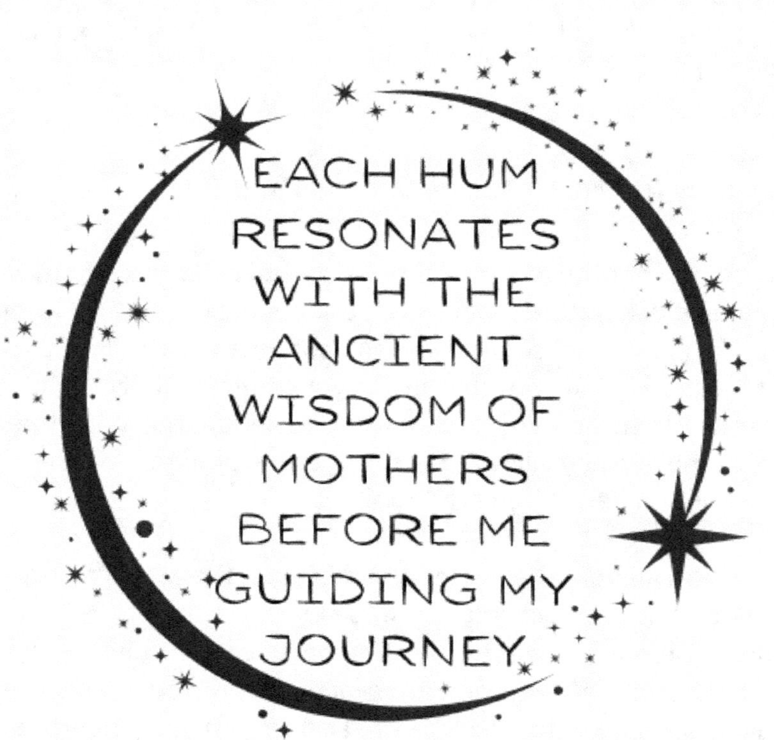
EACH HUM
RESONATES
WITH THE
ANCIENT
WISDOM OF
MOTHERS
BEFORE ME
GUIDING MY
JOURNEY

Five

Active Labor – Riding the Waves with a Hum

Welcome to active labor. This is the part of the process where things start to heat up, where each contraction feels more insistent, like a tidal wave rolling in. You've moved beyond the gentle rhythms of early labor, and now your body is fully committed to this task of bringing life into the world. Here's where humming transforms from a gentle companion to a powerful force—a tool that helps you ride each wave with strength, grace, and a touch of calm.

Active labor can feel intense, no doubt about it. But this is also the moment when your hum comes into its own, when its resonance matches the depth of each contraction. Think of it like a dance partner guiding you, helping you find stability and rhythm even as the waves grow stronger. Let's explore how to use humming to stay grounded, focused, and resilient through this stage.

Amplifying the Hum: Embracing Depth and Strength

As labor progresses, it's natural for your hum to become deeper, fuller, and more intense. At this stage, you might feel drawn to let your hum expand, to give it a little more volume. Don't hold back—let your hum be as big as you need it to be. This isn't about polite sounds; this is about harnessing the raw, primal power of your voice.

Each deep, resonant hum is like a release valve, allowing the intensity of the contraction to move through you instead of getting trapped inside. By humming deeply, you're matching the strength of each wave, giving yourself a powerful outlet to stay grounded. The hum becomes a steady anchor in the midst of labor's intensity, keeping you focused, engaged, and connected.

Syncing Humming with Breath: A Dance of Inhale and Exhale

In active labor, your breathing may naturally pick up pace, becoming shorter and more frequent. This is perfectly normal, but it can also create tension. Humming offers a way to bring intentionality back to your breath, guiding you to find a balanced, rhythmic pattern even in the heat of each contraction.

As a contraction builds, try this: take a deep inhale through your nose, then release it with a long, steady hum. Picture the hum as a bridge, linking the intensity of the contraction with the calm of the exhale. By focusing on your hum, you're not only regulating your breath; you're also signaling to your body that you're safe, that you're present, and that you can handle this.

This dance of inhale and exhale becomes a powerful way to navigate contractions, keeping you centered and helping your body flow with the natural rhythm of labor.

Staying Present: Using Humming as a Focal Point

One of the challenges of active labor is the intensity—it can feel overwhelming, like a rollercoaster ride with no brakes. The hum provides a focal point, something to ground you, even when the waves feel particularly strong. When you feel a contraction coming, let your mind focus solely on the hum. This sound, this vibration, becomes your lifeline.

By concentrating on the sensation of the hum, you're anchoring yourself in the present moment, taking each contraction as it comes rather than getting lost in anticipation. Your mind has somewhere to rest, a place to go that isn't solely wrapped up in the pain or intensity of the experience. The hum becomes a mantra, a way to remind yourself that you are fully present, fully engaged, and fully capable.

Humming and Hormones: A Dance of Oxytocin and Endorphins

In active labor, humming continues to play a role in supporting the release of oxytocin and endorphins. These hormones become even more crucial as labor intensifies, helping to regulate contractions and manage pain. Each hum acts like a gentle nudge to your body, encouraging it to release oxytocin and keep contractions flowing, allowing labor to progress smoothly.

Endorphins, too, are part of this dance. With each hum, you're releasing these natural pain relievers, giving yourself a bit of comfort and resilience in the face of labor's demands. Think of these hormones as your allies, a team of inner helpers brought to life by your own voice. Humming taps into your body's natural capacity for resilience, enhancing your ability to move through each contraction with strength and grace.

The Vibrational Massage: Soothing and Supporting Your Body

At this stage, the physical sensation of the hum becomes even more significant. When you hum deeply, you create a vibration that resonates through your body, almost like an internal massage. This vibration is particularly helpful in active labor, when muscles are working hard, and tension may start to build.

Imagine the hum as a soothing wave moving through your body, releasing areas of tension, helping muscles to relax, and giving your body the support it needs. Whether you're feeling pressure in your back, abdomen, or pelvis, let the hum act as a gentle massage, a way to relieve and soothe each area as you continue through labor.

Embracing the Power: Letting Go of Resistance

Active labor is often where we start to feel the urge to resist, to push back against the intensity. But here's the magic of the hum—it helps you release resistance. When you hum, you're actively inviting each contraction in, working with it instead of against it.

Each hum is a message to your body: "I'm here with you. I'm not resisting." By letting go of resistance, you allow each contraction to do its work, helping labor progress and bringing you one step closer to meeting your baby. The hum becomes a sound of surrender, a way of saying yes to the process, yes to the power, yes to the incredible strength within you.

Moving with Your Hum: Finding Positions That Support Your Sound

As labor progresses, you may feel drawn to different positions—standing, kneeling, rocking, or even leaning forward. The beauty of the hum is that it adapts with you, becoming a companion no matter how you choose to position your body. If you're on your hands and knees, let the hum be low and deep, vibrating down to the core. If you're standing or swaying, let the hum match the rhythm of your movements.

Moving with your hum is like adding another layer to its power. It becomes not only a sound but a rhythm, a movement, a way of connecting with the flow of your body. Each contraction becomes less of an obstacle and more of an invitation, something you can work with, move with, and navigate with confidence.

Staying Grounded, Staying Open

Active labor can be a whirlwind, but it's also a time of tremendous strength, a time to tap into the well of power you've always had. Humming helps you stay grounded, even as the intensity rises. It keeps you open to the process, reminding you that you are safe, that you are strong, and that you are capable of handling whatever comes your way.

Each hum is a moment of connection—a reminder that you are not just enduring this experience; you are shaping it, guiding it, moving with it. Active labor may challenge you, but with your hum as a companion, you are ready to meet each wave, ride each moment, and continue forward with strength and resilience.

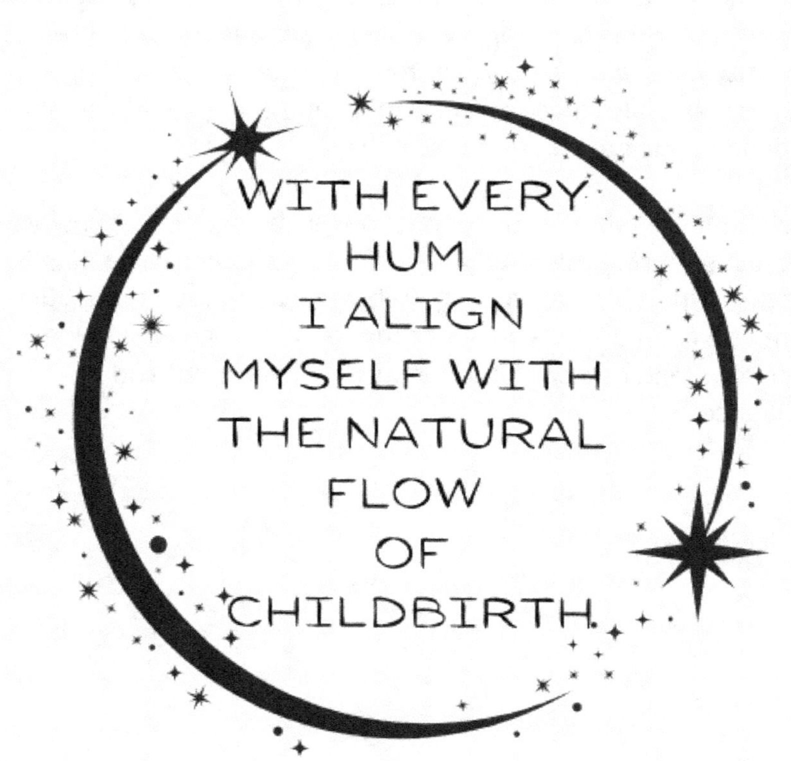
WITH EVERY
HUM
I ALIGN
MYSELF WITH
THE NATURAL
FLOW
OF
CHILDBIRTH.

Six

Transition – The Storm Before the Calm

You've made it this far, humming your way through early and active labor, dancing with each contraction. But here we are at transition—the part of labor known for its intensity, unpredictability, and, let's be honest, a little chaos. This is where things get real. Contractions come fast and fierce, often without much space to catch your breath, and you may feel like you've hit your limit. But transition, as powerful and all-consuming as it can feel, is also a sign that you're nearing the end of this marathon. You're so close to meeting your baby.

Transition is often called the "storm before the calm," and it's where the hum truly becomes a lifeline. When you're feeling stretched to your very edge, this practice will be your anchor. Think of each hum as a lighthouse guiding you through the storm, keeping you grounded and present, even as labor surges forward. Let's explore how to use your hum to move through this stage with courage, resilience, and trust.

Deepening the Hum: Surrendering to the Power of Transition

If active labor felt like riding waves, transition might feel more like braving a storm at sea. The intensity can be overwhelming, and it's common to feel like things are spiraling out of control. But this is where the deep, primal power of your hum can help you let go of resistance and surrender to the process.

When each contraction comes, allow your hum to go even deeper. You may feel the need to let out a longer, louder sound—and that's exactly what transition calls for. By letting your hum mirror the depth and power of each contraction, you're no longer resisting; you're flowing with it. This surrender is one of the most powerful acts of trust, a way of saying to your body, "I'm with you, I'm in this."

Trusting the Process: Humming as a Reminder of Your Strength

Transition can bring up every doubt in the book. You may feel uncertain, even afraid, wondering if you can keep going. This is the moment to let your hum be a reminder of the strength you've built, of everything you've already handled, of every wave you've already ridden. The hum becomes more than a sound—it's a promise to yourself, a reminder that you are capable, resilient, and ready.

Each time you hum, you're grounding yourself in that strength. You're choosing to stay present, to trust your body, to trust the process. Yes, transition is intense, but it's also temporary. With each hum, you're one step closer to the calm, to the moment of release, to the arrival of your baby.

Embracing the Primal: Letting Your Voice Go Where It Needs To

Transition is a raw, primal experience, and so is the hum that accompanies it. This isn't the time for quiet, reserved sounds. This is the time to let your voice go wherever it needs to. If your hum becomes a growl, a low moan, or even a roar, let it happen. The hum is flexible; it will meet you wherever you are.

This is the moment to tune into the ancient wisdom of the body. For centuries, women have been vocalizing through birth, using sound as a way to channel energy, release tension, and stay connected to their power. When you hum in transition, you're connecting to that lineage, drawing on the strength of generations of birthing women. You're tapping into a well of courage and resilience that's far bigger than this moment.

Holding On When It Feels Like Too Much

It's completely normal to feel like transition is too much—that the contractions are too intense, too close together, too overwhelming. This is a common experience, and it doesn't mean you're not strong enough; it just means you're human. The hum can be a lifeline here, giving you something steady to hold onto when the world feels shaky.

When a contraction hits and feels unbearable, close your eyes, take a deep breath, and release it with the longest, deepest hum you can muster. Focus all your energy on that sound, letting it be your anchor. Even if everything around you feels chaotic, that hum is a place of stability, a reminder that you're still here, that you're still breathing, that you're still moving forward.

The Hormonal Surge: Riding the Wave of Oxytocin and Adrenaline

Transition is the stage when your body releases a powerful cocktail of hormones—oxytocin and adrenaline—that intensifies contractions and prepares you for the final push. Oxytocin strengthens contractions, while adrenaline sharpens your senses, getting you ready for the moment of birth. This surge can feel overwhelming, like an inner storm, but humming helps you ride it out, grounding you even as your body ramps up for what's next.

The hum supports your body's natural rhythms, keeping you steady and calm in the midst of the hormonal rush. Each hum signals to your brain and body that you're safe, that you're strong, that you're in control. By humming through transition, you're not just coping with the intensity—you're aligning with it, allowing it to carry you forward.

Using Humming as a Mental Anchor: Finding Presence in the Storm

The mind can be a tricky place during transition. This is the stage when thoughts of doubt, fear, or self-criticism can creep in. It's also when you might feel the urge to disconnect, to mentally check out because it all feels too intense. But here's the beauty of humming—it keeps you present.

By focusing on the hum, you're giving your mind a place to land, a point of concentration that keeps you engaged. Let the hum be your meditation, your mantra, your constant companion. Each sound is an affirmation of your ability to stay present, even when things get challenging. It's a reminder that you are fully in this experience, that you are capable, that you are in harmony with your body's natural process.

Hummingbirth

Finding the Calm Within the Intensity

Transition can feel all-consuming, but within the storm, there is always a center of calm. This calm doesn't mean the contractions are any less intense; it means that you've found a place within yourself that is steady, a place that is connected to something deeper. Humming helps you access that center, even as labor reaches its peak.

When you hum, imagine that calmness spreading through your body, like a warm light expanding from your core. Each contraction is a wave, but you are the steady shore. Each hum is a reminder of that stability, that inner strength that cannot be shaken. You are not just riding the storm—you are part of it, fully grounded, fully present.

Honoring Your Power

Transition is the part of labor that asks you to tap into a power you may not have known you had. It's raw, it's intense, and yes, it's challenging. But humming through transition allows you to harness that power, to feel it in every cell of your being. Each hum is a testament to your courage, a reminder that you are doing something extraordinary, that you are embracing the fullness of this experience.

As you hum through the final contractions, know that you are honoring your body, your baby, and yourself. You are embodying the strength, resilience, and beauty of birth. This is your power, your process, your sound. Transition may be intense, but it is also the bridge to the calm, to the release, to the moment when you'll meet your baby.

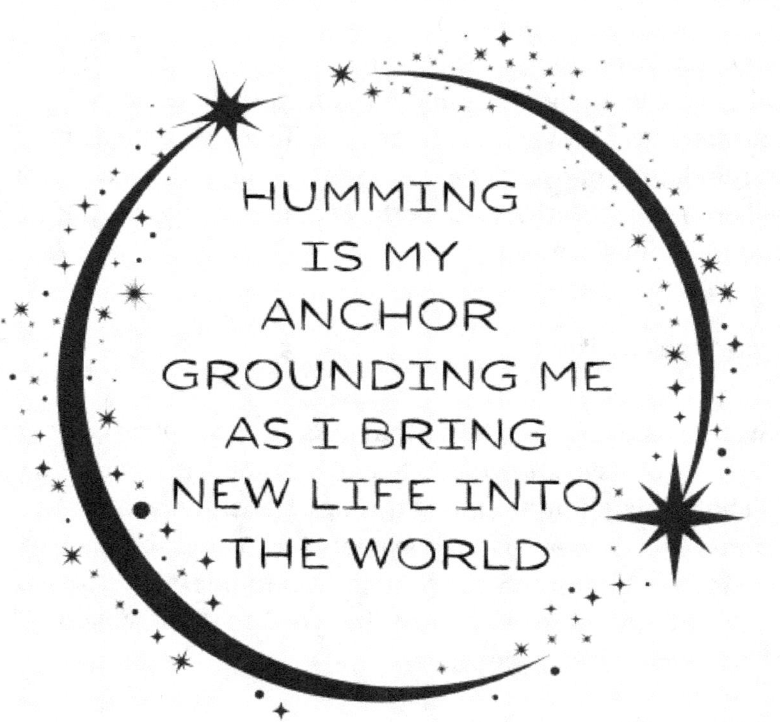
HUMMING
IS MY
ANCHOR
GROUNDING ME
AS I BRING
NEW LIFE INTO
THE WORLD

Seven

The Pushing Stage – The Power of Sound and Strength

Here we are, the final stage of labor: pushing. This is the moment you've been working toward, humming through the waves, riding out the intensity, holding steady through transition. Now, your body is shifting into an entirely different gear—one that brings you face-to-face with the full force of your power. If earlier stages were about letting go, this one is about summoning strength, about channeling your energy with purpose. Here, the hum shifts too, from a steady companion to a call to action, a rallying cry.

Let's talk about how humming can support you in the pushing stage, helping you bring every ounce of your strength and focus to the surface.

Channeling Energy: From Release to Power

In the earlier stages, humming was a way to let go, to flow with each contraction and ride out the intensity. But now, in this stage, humming takes on a different role. This isn't about relaxing; it's about focusing. It's about gathering all the strength you've cultivated, all the energy you've conserved, and directing it toward the work of bringing your baby into the world.

Think of each hum now as a way to harness and concentrate your energy. Let your hum be shorter, stronger, even sharper if that feels right. The sound can match the effort of each push, grounding you, focusing you, connecting you to the deep reserves of power within your body. You're no longer just moving with the rhythm of labor—you're actively shaping it, steering it, using it.

Vocalizing with Intention: Allowing Your Voice to Guide Each Push

During the pushing stage, you may feel an instinct to vocalize in new ways. Some women find themselves grunting, groaning, or making sounds that come from a place deeper than words—a primal expression of the body's power and intensity. This is your body speaking, telling you what it needs, guiding you through each push.

Let your hum become whatever it needs to be—louder, rougher, more forceful. If it shifts into a roar or a deep groan, embrace it. Sound is one of the most natural ways to release tension, to tap into energy, to give your body a focal point for all the effort you're pouring into each push. By vocalizing, you're not just expressing your strength; you're amplifying it, guiding it, letting it flow.

The Physiology of Pushing: Humming to Stay Calm and Focused

During pushing, your body releases a final surge of oxytocin, which not only strengthens contractions but also deepens your sense of connection with your baby. Humming helps keep you focused and calm in the midst of this intense experience, grounding you even as your body shifts into full action mode.

Think of your hum as a reminder to stay present and breathe through each push. As you inhale deeply, feel the air filling your lungs, and as you exhale with a hum, let that sound ground you. This rhythm of breath and hum helps keep your nervous system steady, even as the work of pushing demands all your energy and attention. It's easy to get caught up in the effort, to hold your breath, to strain. But humming brings you back to a steady rhythm, keeping your focus on breathing and pacing each push.

Hummingbirth

Finding Your Rhythm: Letting the Hum Lead You Through Each Push

Pushing can sometimes feel like a series of start-and-stop efforts, and that can be frustrating. You're giving everything you've got, and it's easy to feel like each push should be "it"—the one that brings your baby to you. But the pushing stage has its own rhythm, one that builds gradually, with each push bringing you a little closer.

Humming can help you find a sustainable rhythm, giving each push its own sense of purpose without depleting you. Try humming as you bear down with each contraction, feeling the hum as a steady, even pulse that supports your efforts. This rhythm helps you stay focused without losing your energy. Each hum becomes a reminder that progress is being made, that you're moving forward, even if it's only one small step at a time.

Embracing the Primal Power: Letting Go of Inhibitions

The pushing stage can bring out a side of you that may surprise you. This is the moment when inhibitions fall away, when you tap into a primal power that goes beyond thought, beyond language, beyond everyday experience. This is raw, unapologetic strength, and it may feel intense, overwhelming, even out of control.

Let the hum support you in this primal space. Don't hold back. Let your sound become as fierce, as bold, as powerful as it needs to be. This is not a time to stay quiet or reserved. This is your body working at its peak, your voice expressing the depths of that power. Embrace it, let it guide you, let it connect you to every woman who has ever brought life into the world.

Hummingbirth

Humming as Connection: Building the Bond with Your Baby

In the midst of this intense stage, it's easy to focus on the physical demands, to lose sight of the incredible connection that's forming with your baby. But humming brings you back to that bond, reminding you that each push is bringing you closer to holding your child.

As you hum through each push, imagine that sound traveling down to your baby, a way of communicating, a way of guiding them forward. The hum becomes a sound of connection, a reminder that you and your baby are in this together, that each push is a step closer to meeting each other face-to-face.

Releasing into the Final Push

As you near the end of the pushing stage, you may feel a mix of excitement, exhaustion, and even disbelief. The finish line is so close, but every push feels monumental. Let your hum be the sound that carries you through, that encourages you to give just a little bit more, to trust that you have everything you need to see this through.

When the final push comes, you may feel an instinct to release everything, to let out one final, powerful hum that encapsulates the whole journey. This release is not just physical; it's emotional, it's spiritual, it's the culmination of every wave, every contraction, every moment of strength and surrender.

In that moment, your hum is a sound of triumph, a sound of completion, a sound that welcomes your baby into the world.

Hummingbirth

With the end of this chapter, the hum has taken on its fullest expression: it has been your guide, your companion, your power, and your release. Each sound has brought you closer to your baby, carrying you through the entire journey of labor and birth. As you enter the next stage—holding your newborn—your voice may quiet, but the hum's impact will remain, a part of the connection you've built with yourself and with the new life in your arms.

Please STOP and Review this book!

Your Voice Matters

If this book has resonated with you—brought you insight, comfort, or a sense of possibility—please consider leaving a review. Reviews aren't just for me (though I'll cherish every word). They're a lifeline for the mother searching for hope in the stillness of the night, for the midwife longing for a gentler way, and for the women who haven't yet discovered how transformative birth can be.

Your words can help this message reach more women, creating a ripple effect of empowerment and change. When we change the way we birth, we change the way we live—and that's the kind of revolution worth humming about.

Eight

Real Life Birth Stories – The Hum in Action

Theories, techniques, and science are all valuable, but there's something powerful about hearing real stories—moments when the hum became not just a technique but a trusted friend, a source of strength, a calming balm in the midst of labor. These are stories from women who've walked this path, who've used the Hummingbirth method to navigate their unique journeys. Each story is different, each birth an experience all its own, but together they show how the hum can be a transformative tool in labor.

Whether these mothers were at home, in a hospital, or anywhere in between, their stories reveal how humming helped them find calm in chaos, power in vulnerability, and joy in the unexpected. Here are a few of their stories.

Story 1: Sarah's Surprise – Finding Calm Through the Storm

Sarah had planned a home birth, wanting the familiarity of her own space and the support of her partner and midwife. But at 38 weeks, her water broke, and she went into labor fast and furiously. As soon as the contractions started, they were intense and close together, leaving her little time to catch her breath.

"I remember feeling totally overwhelmed at first," Sarah said. "It felt like I was thrown into the deep end without any warning."

Her midwife suggested she start humming, something Sarah had practiced but hadn't expected to need so soon. As each contraction came, she closed her eyes, took a deep breath, and released a long, low hum.

"It was like flipping a switch. Suddenly, I had something to hold onto," she explained. "Each hum became this little moment of calm, a way to slow everything down. I wasn't focusing on the pain—I was just focusing on my breath, my sound. The hum made me feel like I was in control, even though the labor was moving fast."

Sarah's labor lasted just five hours, and she credits humming for helping her stay grounded and calm through every intense contraction. "I truly don't know how I would have managed without it," she said. "It helped me stay present, and I think that's why my labor felt so empowering, even though it was way faster than I'd expected."

Story 2: Lily's Hospital Birth – A Tool for Peace and Privacy

Lily had chosen a hospital birth, wanting the reassurance of medical support. She'd practiced the Hummingbirth method during her pregnancy, seeing it as a way to feel more in control and less fearful of the birth process. As her labor progressed, she found herself surrounded by a steady stream of nurses, doctors, and equipment, and at times it felt overwhelming.

"When I started humming, it was like creating this bubble around myself," Lily said. "I could tune out all the noises, all the people coming in and out. It felt like it was just me and my baby."

Lily's hums were soft and steady, a quiet vibration that helped her feel centered. The hum gave her a sense of peace and privacy, even in the middle of a bustling hospital room.

"I remember one nurse came over and started humming with me," Lily laughed. "It was like she just understood that this was my space, my little world. By the time I was pushing, the whole room was quieter, like everyone was respecting the calm I'd created with my hum."

Lily's labor was long but smooth, and she delivered a healthy baby girl. Looking back, she sees humming as her anchor, a way to stay present and grounded in a place where she initially felt out of place. "It was the hum that kept me connected to myself," she said. "I didn't feel lost or overwhelmed. I felt in control."

Story 3: Maya's Unexpected Twist – Embracing the Power of the Hum

Maya had practiced the Hummingbirth method but wasn't sure how effective it would be. When her labor began, everything seemed manageable. She was at home with her doula, her partner was by her side, and she felt confident. But as her labor progressed, it became clear that her baby was positioned "sunny side up" (occiput posterior), meaning the back of the baby's head was pressing on her spine.

"The back pain was like nothing I'd ever felt," Maya recalled. "I was in tears, wondering if I could really do this."

Her doula encouraged her to lean into the hum, to let each sound help her release the tension and find comfort, even if only for a moment. Maya began humming deeply, focusing on letting the vibration move through her lower back, visualizing the sound soothing the pain.

"It didn't take the pain away," she admitted, "but it gave me a way to cope with it. Every hum felt like a release, like I was breathing out some of the pain instead of holding onto it."

Hours later, Maya delivered her baby, feeling a mix of relief and amazement. She'd faced one of the hardest labors she could imagine, but the hum had been her companion, her source of strength. "I don't think I would have had the same experience without the hum. It helped me find peace in a really painful, difficult labor. I felt like I could handle anything."

Story 4: Emma's First-Time Birth – Using Humming to Replace Fear

Emma, a first-time mom, had always been nervous about giving birth. She'd heard countless stories of long, painful labors and was terrified that she wouldn't be able to cope. She found the Hummingbirth method through a friend and decided to give it a try, seeing it as a way to manage her anxiety and feel more prepared.

When her labor began, she felt the familiar wave of fear start to creep in, but she remembered the humming practice and started with a gentle hum.

"Every time I felt afraid, I would just hum," Emma said. "The sound was like a warm blanket around me. It felt safe."

As labor progressed, Emma continued humming, letting each sound calm her mind and focus her attention. She found herself entering a rhythm, where fear melted away, replaced by the hum's steady reassurance.

"I didn't feel afraid anymore. I felt like I was in control, that I had a tool that no one could take away from me."

Emma's labor was smooth and steady, and she delivered her baby after eight hours. She describes the experience as "transformative," a journey that took her from fear to empowerment. "The hum was more than just a sound," she said. "It was my way of saying, 'I can do this. I'm not afraid.'"

Hummingbirth

Story 5: Angela's Water Birth – A Harmonious Rhythm

Angela had always dreamed of a water birth, picturing the calm, soothing environment as the perfect setting for her labor. She'd practiced the Hummingbirth method religiously, hoping to use it as her main form of pain management.

As she labored in the warm water, Angela began humming with each contraction, finding a gentle, harmonious rhythm that matched the water's movement.

"It felt like I was floating, like my hum was part of the water," Angela recalled. "Every contraction became a wave, and the hum was my way of moving with it."

Angela's water birth was peaceful and empowering, a labor experience that felt almost like a meditation. "The hum helped me stay connected to the water, to my body, to my baby. It was like we were all moving together."

Angela's baby arrived smoothly, born into an atmosphere of calm and peace. Looking back, Angela sees the Hummingbirth method as a perfect complement to the water birth she'd envisioned. "The hum was my rhythm," she said. "It made my birth feel like a beautiful dance."

Each of these stories shows a different journey, a different challenge, a different labor experience. But in each case, the hum was there—a steady guide, a trusted companion, a powerful tool. These women's experiences illustrate the flexibility and effectiveness of the Hummingbirth method, proving that no matter what kind of labor you face, the hum can support you, ground you, and empower you.

As you prepare for your own birth, know that the hum is ready to be part of your story too. It can meet you wherever you are, adapt to whatever you need, and carry you through each moment of your journey. Let these stories inspire you, comfort you, and remind you that you have a powerful, timeless tool at your fingertips—one that women have used for generations to bring life into the world.

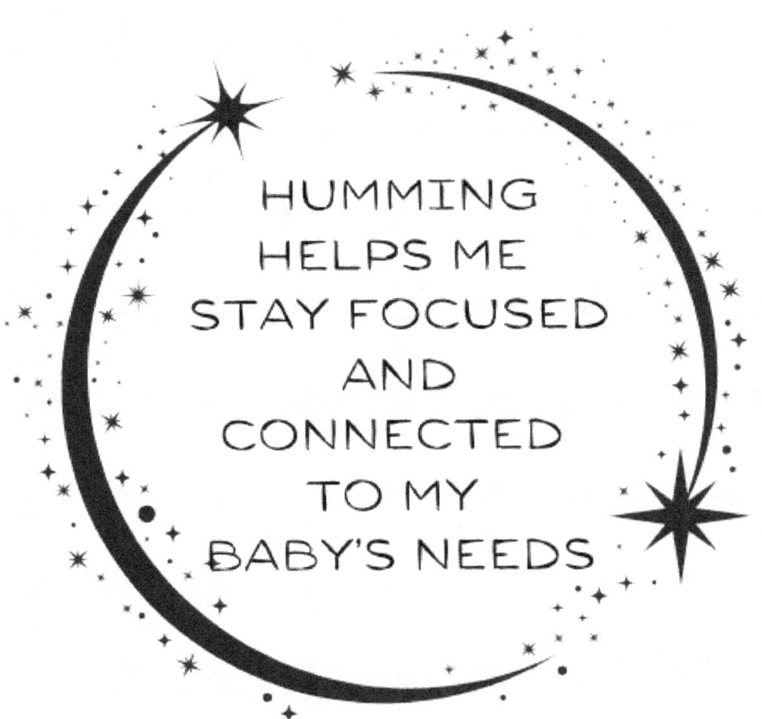
HUMMING
HELPS ME
STAY FOCUSED
AND
CONNECTED
TO MY
BABY'S NEEDS

Nine

The Role of Partners – Humming in Harmony

Let's talk about the people standing by you when things get real. Partners. The ones who promised to be there when it was all abstract and hypothetical, who said, "Of course I'll be there! I'll do whatever you need!" And here we are, getting very literal about what you need. A partner in birth is like the percussion section of an orchestra: subtle, steady, keeps the beat, and, ideally, doesn't take over with their own solo.

You may not know exactly what role you want your partner to play right now—mostly because it's hard to imagine until you're actually there. But there's something grounding about having someone who's committed to being by your side, even if they're fumbling with water bottles and mistiming shoulder rubs. And now, lucky for them, they get to learn the fine art of humming along with you.

The Sympathetic Hum: Finding Their Sound

Here's where partners come in. Maybe they're going to hum along with you, maybe they're going to hum softly at a respectful distance, or maybe they'll just listen to you like they're in an intimate concert. Humming can actually be a fantastic way for your partner to support you without saying too much or too little. And if they're humming too, they're activating that vagus nerve and calming themselves down as well—essential if things start to feel tense.

Consider this: when a partner hums with you, they're actively doing something. It's a simple, concrete way for them to contribute to the calm, to show up in the moment with you.

Think of it as an invitation to sync up, to find a rhythm together. And maybe, if things start to feel a bit intense or overwhelming, their hum becomes the calm that steadies you, the sound you can latch onto when you're deep in the zone.

Support Over Spectacle

Now, let's talk about roles. The best birth partners are the ones who are steady and encouraging, but not starring in their own drama. This isn't about their nerves or how well they think they're doing at "being supportive." Their job is to make sure you feel safe and unobserved, like you're in a little bubble of calm, and yes, occasionally to bring you ice chips or a back rub without fanfare.

A partner can be your anchor—a physical and emotional touchstone who keeps you grounded and reminds you that you're not alone. They don't need to recite motivational speeches or rub your shoulders in perfect rhythm with each contraction. They just need to be there, quietly supporting, ready to offer whatever you need without a lot of fuss.

A Symphony of Breaths and Beats

Humming together isn't just a nice idea; it's scientifically backed, too. Studies suggest that couples who are in sync—who breathe together, hum together, move together—create a kind of harmony that can actually help manage stress and pain. When both of you are humming, you're not only engaging in the birth process together, but you're literally creating vibrations that resonate with each other. You're sending each other silent messages of, "I'm here, you're here, we're doing this together."

And don't worry if your partner is "tone-deaf" or feels self-conscious. This isn't a performance. In fact, the stranger their hum sounds, the more endearing it may feel in the moment. It's just another layer of connection, a reminder that they're there, in this very real, very raw experience with you.

Giving the Partner Permission to Be a Goof

One more thing. This journey is serious and important, yes, but a little humor never hurts. Partners, this is your chance to lighten the mood when the time is right, to bring in a little levity when it feels safe. Maybe they offer a little hum remix, maybe they let out a laugh in an otherwise tense moment. The right bit of silliness can sometimes break the tension just enough for you both to breathe a little easier.

And in those moments when things feel downright surreal—when you're deep in the hum, in a world of waves and vibrations, and your partner is humming like a meditational monk in the background—let yourselves smile at the absurdity of it all. Here you both are, making sounds you might never have made before, diving into this ancient, primal dance of bringing a new life into the world.

When You Need Them, They're There

The point is, your partner doesn't have to be perfect or polished. They just need to be present, in whatever way is most supportive to you. And humming—humming with you, for you, or even just nearby—is one of the simplest, most profound ways they can do that. Whether they're a natural born hummer or nervously trying it out for the first time, their hum is a part of the symphony you're creating together, a steady note in the harmony of this shared experience.

Hummingbirth

So to all the partners reading this, go ahead, find your hum.
Embrace it. Let it be your way of anchoring, of grounding, of
being the safe and steady sound that carries your loved one
through. Because in this beautiful, unpredictable, transformative
dance of birth, sometimes the most powerful thing you can do is
simply be there—humming your heart out.

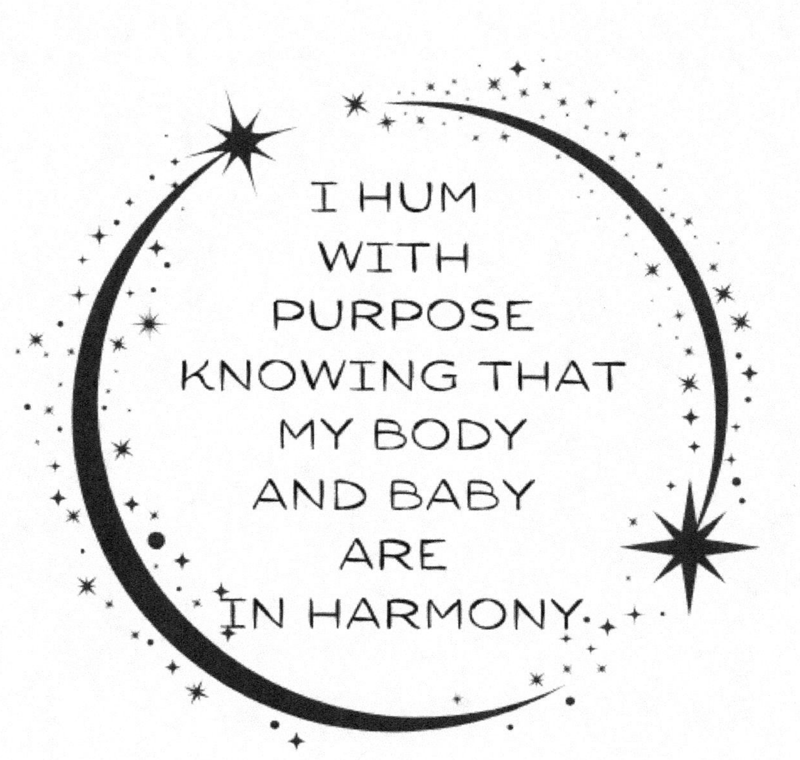

I HUM
WITH
PURPOSE
KNOWING THAT
MY BODY
AND BABY
ARE
IN HARMONY.

Ten

Frequently Asked Questions – The Hum, Unraveled

Ah, the questions. There's no shortage of them, and they're all good. In fact, if you didn't have questions, I'd be worried. Birth is a monumental journey, and when it comes to humming through it, you may wonder about everything from logistics to the science behind it. So here's a collection of frequently asked questions about the Hummingbirth method, answered with the care, wit, and no-nonsense practicality you deserve.

Q: Do I have to hum out loud, or can I hum in my head?

A: I get it—maybe you're picturing yourself humming in a crowded hospital room and feeling, well, a little awkward. But here's the truth: the magic lies in the sound *and* the vibration. When you hum aloud, you're creating actual physical vibrations that activate your vagus nerve, which can calm your system and even ease pain. The hum in your head is lovely for, say, waiting rooms or awkward elevator rides, but the real benefits come when you let that sound out.

Q: What if I'm tone-deaf? Will my hum still work?

A: Absolutely, yes. This is not about getting on "The Voice." Humming for birth is as much about the vibration as it is about the sound, so even if your hum is slightly off-key or sounds more like a lawnmower than a lullaby, it's still doing its job. Your body doesn't care about pitch; it cares about vibration, and the hum will work as long as you keep at it.

Hummingbirth

Q: Is humming really a pain reliever?

A: I know—it sounds almost too simple to be true, but yes, humming can genuinely help manage pain. When you hum, you release endorphins, which are your body's natural painkillers. You also activate that fabulous vagus nerve, which tells your body to chill out a bit, calming your heart rate, blood pressure, and reducing your perception of pain. Think of it as a low-tech, high-impact tool that your body is already primed to respond to.

Q: Will people think I'm a little "out there" if I hum through labor?

A: Perhaps. But here's the thing: giving birth is about you and your baby, not the opinions of the hospital staff or your second cousin's girlfriend who happens to be in the waiting room. By the time you're really in the zone, you probably won't care anyway. You're humming because it helps you, and that's all that matters. Besides, plenty of people use vocalization in labor, so really, you're just taking it to the next (quieter, gentler) level.

Q: How loud should I hum?

A: Loud enough that you feel the vibration, but not so loud that you feel like you're yelling. Imagine you're singing to yourself in the shower—loud enough to fill your own little space, but not quite an aria. The goal is to feel that hum resonate in your chest, your face, maybe even all the way down to your toes.

Q: Can I practice humming with my partner?

A: Yes! In fact, I highly recommend it. Practicing together can help your partner understand the rhythm and effect of the hum, and when they're familiar with it, they're more likely to jump in and hum alongside you during labor. Plus, it's a sweet way to bond and get a little giggle out of your "birth prep karaoke."

Q: What if I forget to hum in the middle of a contraction?

A: Don't sweat it. Labor is not about perfection, and no one's grading you on your humming frequency. You might skip a contraction, or even a few, and that's okay. Just pick up the hum again when you're ready. It's not about being "on" every single second; it's about finding a rhythm that feels natural to you.

Q: I'm nervous I'll forget all of this when labor actually starts. Any tips?

A: Totally normal. A good way to remember is to practice humming whenever you feel stressed in the weeks leading up to your due date. Stuck in traffic? Hum. Feeling anxious about the nursery wallpaper? Hum. It doesn't have to be a big production—just get used to using it as a calming tool. Then, when labor begins, it'll feel like second nature.

Q: Is humming a replacement for pain medication?

A: Not necessarily. Humming is a fantastic, natural pain management tool, and for some women, it's all they need. But labor is unpredictable, and there's no one right way to get through it. Think of humming as a powerful option in your toolkit. If you choose to use medication, you can still hum along with it! This is about giving yourself options, not taking anything away.

Hummingbirth

Q: Can I hum while I push?

A: Yes, you can! Humming during pushing can help you stay focused and keep your breathing steady. Some women find that it even eases the sensation of pressure. The key is to find a hum that feels natural in the moment. You might be surprised how grounding it is to have a sound to rely on, even when you're summoning all your energy to meet your baby.

Q: Can I hum in between contractions, or is it just for the intense parts?

A: You can absolutely hum in between contractions. In fact, many women find that humming in between contractions helps them stay relaxed and keeps the flow going. Birth is a journey with its own rhythm, and sometimes keeping a low, gentle hum throughout can create a feeling of continuous calm.

Q: What if I don't want to hum at all?

A: Fair question! If humming doesn't feel right for you, that's okay. The goal is for you to feel calm and empowered, so if you find another technique that resonates more with you, go for it. But I'd still recommend giving the hum a shot; it may feel odd at first, but many women are surprised by how effective it can be.

Q: Can humming help during other times of stress, not just labor?

A: Absolutely. Humming isn't just a birth tool—it's a life tool. It can help calm nerves, refocus your mind, and bring you back to center in almost any situation. So feel free to hum your way through dentist appointments, job interviews, or anytime you need a little extra calm.

Q: I have no idea how I'll actually feel when I'm in labor. Will humming still work if I'm nervous or panicked?

A: Here's the thing: humming is designed to help *with* the nerves and the panic. When you're anxious, the vibrations of the hum can activate your body's relaxation response, calming your heart rate and telling your system to ease up on the tension. So even if you start out feeling nervous, give humming a try. You may be surprised at how much it can help.

Q: Okay, but is there any downside to humming during labor?

A: Honestly? None that I've ever encountered. It doesn't cost anything, requires no special equipment, and is entirely under your control. The worst that could happen is maybe your throat gets a little scratchy, or you decide that it's not your thing. In that case, you can let it go and try something else. But you might just find that humming becomes a quiet, beautiful part of your birth story.

Hummingbirth

Q: Can I hum and curse at the same time?

A: Funny you should ask! Labor is a full-contact sport, and there's room for all the sounds you need. If humming for ten minutes straight and then letting out a curse or two makes you feel better, then by all means, hum and curse in harmony. This is your birth, your soundscape. Don't hold back.

And there you have it. The hum, unraveled. Every question is fair game here, and there's no right or wrong way to hum your way through labor. The goal is to feel supported, empowered, and tuned in to what you and your body need. So go forth with your hum, however it works for you, knowing that you have one more beautiful, calming, powerful tool to lean on as you welcome this new life into the world.

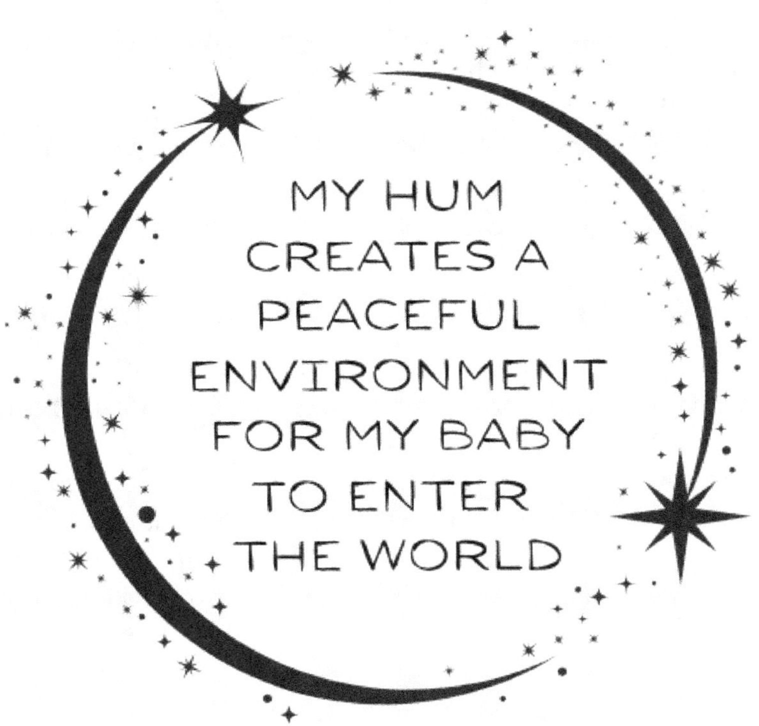
MY HUM
CREATES A
PEACEFUL
ENVIRONMENT
FOR MY BABY
TO ENTER
THE WORLD

Eleven

Making Humming Part of Your Pregnancy Journey – Preparing for Labor and Beyond

So here we are, with the hum now firmly in your birth toolbox, nestled between your birth playlist and that half-joking, half-serious list of "must-have" snacks for the hospital bag. Humming may seem like a small thing, but it's a technique you can use well beyond the delivery room. Here's how you can start incorporating humming into your pregnancy routine now, so by the time you're in labor, it feels as natural as reaching for a deep breath or holding someone's hand.

The Prenatal Hum

Think of this as a warm-up phase. You don't wait until a marathon to put on your running shoes and hope for the best; you train a little. The same goes for humming. You don't have to dedicate hours to it, but take some time each week to hum, to get used to the vibrations, the rhythm, and the calm that it brings. You'll be practicing the fine art of relaxing on cue, and by the time labor rolls around, you'll have this calmness built into your muscle memory.

Choose moments throughout your day to hum: in the car, in the shower, or while waiting for the water to boil. At first, it may feel a bit odd—like talking to yourself in public or singing "Happy Birthday" alone. But keep at it. Eventually, it will feel like the natural response to moments of stress, or even just when you want to settle in and be present.

Building the Habit

Hummingbirth

Here's a little secret: habit-building with humming is actually pretty easy. Unlike the kind of routines that require willpower, like reminding yourself to drink 12 glasses of water or walk 10,000 steps, humming is something you can do anytime, anywhere. Once you experience how good it feels, it tends to reinforce itself.

Think of times in your day when you're feeling rushed, frazzled, or just plain annoyed. Stuck in traffic? Hum. Waiting in line? Hum. Hear a song you like on the radio? Hum along. Notice how, even in non-stressful moments, humming brings you into the moment, quiets your thoughts, and creates a sense of presence. You're building a pathway to calm that you can follow when labor arrives.

Making It Part of Prenatal Care

You know those breathing exercises and prenatal yoga classes you've heard so much about? Humming can slide right in there. In fact, if you're already doing yoga or deep breathing, humming is an ideal complement. While you're sitting in child's pose or practicing slow breathing, add a hum on the exhale. Close your eyes, tune into the vibration, and imagine it reaching every corner of your body.

At the close Aof this book, you'll discover a link to a guided humming meditation series and a downloadable PDF of humming affirmations—crafted lovingly, just for you. These tools are meant to slip seamlessly into the rhythm of your days, weaving through your pregnancy and into the wider expanse of your life. May they bring more peace, joy, and confidence to your personal journey.

Tuning in with Baby

Let's talk about the star of the show—your baby. From about 18-20 weeks, your baby's sense of hearing starts to develop, and by the time they're born, they're already tuned into the sound of your voice. When you hum, those vibrations reach your baby, surrounding them in a gentle, soothing sound that can bring calm to you both.

Think of it as your first lullaby—a little sound ritual between the two of you. As you hum, take a moment to imagine your baby hearing and feeling the soft vibrations. In the months to come, this hum will become a touchstone, a sound that's tied to a deep sense of calm for both you and your little one.

The Third Trimester Tune-Up

Now that you're getting closer to labor, you might feel the stakes rising a bit. Things are starting to feel real, maybe a little surreal. This is the perfect time to take your humming practice up a notch. At this stage, your hum can become an anchor, a sound that grounds you and reminds you that you've got tools at your disposal.

When those third-trimester jitters come up—the worries about birth, the "am I ready?" moments—lean into the hum. You've practiced it so well that now it's second nature, a way to calm the mind and body together. You're no longer just humming to relax; you're humming as part of your toolkit, part of your plan.

Postpartum Humming

This is the part where people sometimes forget to take care of themselves, where all the energy is funneled into this tiny, beautiful new person who takes up all the room in your heart. But here's the thing: the hum can be your ally even after the birth.

When you're exhausted, when you're up in the middle of the night, or when your patience feels thinner than you thought possible, take a deep breath and hum. It's like giving yourself permission to come back to center, to slow down for just a second. And here's a bonus—humming is still soothing for your baby. They've heard it for months, remember?

Hold them close, hum softly, and feel how it calms both of you. It's a simple but powerful reminder that you have resources within you, that this journey is about taking care of you, too.

Making Humming Your Own

The beauty of humming is that it's entirely yours. You don't have to do it a certain way, there are no wrong notes or prescribed rhythms. You might hum in harmony with a song or go completely rogue with your own tune. You might hum softly, or let it ring out loud and strong. It's up to you.

If you're feeling creative, make a playlist of songs you enjoy humming along to. Try a few different types of music— something soft, something upbeat, maybe even something a little silly. Find the hum that feels like home to you, the one that brings a smile or a sense of peace.

The Hum as Legacy

Remember, the hum isn't just a tool for birth; it's a legacy you're creating for you and your child. This simple sound that you've practiced and learned can stay with you both, a little bit of wisdom passed down from your body to theirs. The rhythm, the calm, the presence—it all goes into this shared hum.

Someday, maybe you'll tell your child how you hummed together even before they were born. Maybe they'll find themselves humming to calm their nerves, to soothe their own children, to create a little pocket of peace. The hum has always been a part of us, a simple, beautiful sound that carries us through the big moments and the small. And now, you get to carry it with you, to create this new chapter, hum by hum.

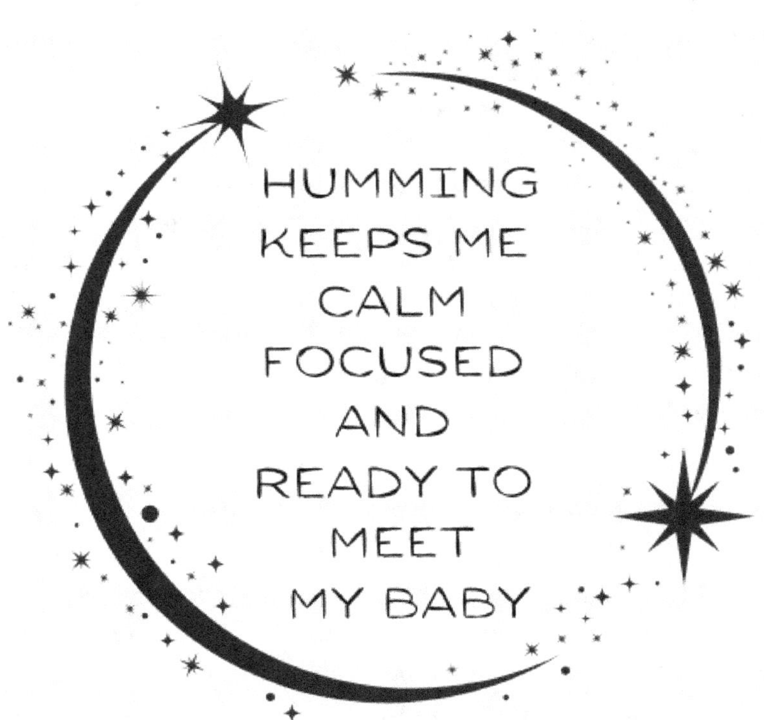

HUMMING
KEEPS ME
CALM
FOCUSED
AND
READY TO
MEET
MY BABY

Twelve

Beyond Birth – How Humming Can Benefit Your Postpartum Recovery

Let's talk about the "other side." The part they don't tell you much about in birth classes, where the spotlight shifts and suddenly it's not about you and your labor journey anymore. Now it's all about this little person who, even as you read this, may be blowing bubbles or squirming in a way that's both adorable and, let's face it, exhausting.

Here's the beautiful, messy truth about postpartum: the ride is not over. Your body is healing, your hormones are doing a tango with your emotions, and sleep? It feels like a fond memory from some other life. But what if I told you that humming could still be there for you, just like it was in labor? You've already learned the power of a well-placed hum—now, let's carry it over into this next phase.

Humming for Emotional Recovery

Ah, the "baby blues." It's a term that makes it sound like a minor inconvenience, like a rainy Tuesday. But for many new mothers, those emotional swings feel a bit more like a tidal wave. Here's where humming comes in handy, with its grounding vibrations and calming effects.

When you're feeling overwhelmed, try humming softly. Science tells us that vocalizing triggers the release of oxytocin and endorphins, those happy little chemicals that can lift your mood and calm your mind. It's a self-soothing tool, and it's something you can do anywhere—while feeding, while rocking, while wondering if you'll ever sleep more than three hours in a row again.

Hummingbirth

A New Spin on the Vagus Nerve

Remember our friend, the vagus nerve, from Chapter 1? That superstar nerve that does everything from lowering blood pressure to helping you feel calm? It's still here for you, still waiting to do its magic. When you hum, you're essentially giving the vagus nerve a gentle nudge, signaling your body to slip into that relaxed state that was so helpful during labor.

Now, in this postpartum time, it's the same effect, just with different benefits. Humming helps your body and mind switch from "all systems go" to "take it easy," even if it's just for a moment. When you hum, you're lowering your cortisol, easing tension, and sending the message to your body that it can start to heal.

Humming as a Focus Tool

Let's be honest—sometimes in the early postpartum days, it feels like your thoughts are scattered across a thousand lists and worries. "Did I order those nursing pads?" "Is that noise normal?" "Is my mother-in-law coming over again?" It's hard to find focus in a brain running on caffeine and hope.

Enter humming as a simple focal point. When you feel that mental chatter creeping up, close your eyes, take a deep breath, and hum. Even a quick, five-second hum can serve as a little reset button, giving your mind something to latch onto. It's a way of quieting the noise, if only for a moment. And sometimes, a moment is all you need.

Physical Recovery and Humming

The weeks after birth are often called the "fourth trimester" for a reason—your body is still doing an incredible amount of work. From shrinking your uterus to healing muscles that worked overtime, it's all happening, even if it's behind the scenes. Humming might feel subtle, but those vibrations aren't just in your head.

When you hum, you're sending those little waves of sound throughout your chest and abdomen. They might be gentle, but they encourage circulation, helping to increase blood flow to healing tissues. It's like giving your muscles and organs a soft, invisible massage, urging them to mend in their own time.

And don't forget, every time you hum, you're breathing deeply, drawing more oxygen into your body—a valuable resource for healing. Humming, with its rhythm and relaxation, can make it easier to take those deep, rejuvenating breaths that your body craves right now.

Bonding with Your Baby

Here's a little surprise: your humming might be the sweetest lullaby your baby has ever heard. After all, they've been hearing that sound for months, and now it's familiar, almost like a heartbeat. When you hum while holding them, you're creating a cocoon of sound and comfort, one that they naturally associate with safety.

Think of it as your very first duet, a simple harmony between you and your little one. It doesn't have to be fancy, and it doesn't even have to make sense. Just hum in those quiet moments, as you're feeding or rocking them. You're not just soothing them;

you're also reinforcing that sense of calm and connection for yourself.

Creating a Personal Humming Ritual

Let's make it official—a little humming ritual just for you. Take a few moments each day, maybe during the quiet of early morning or when everyone else has settled down. Close your eyes, breathe, and hum. This isn't just about self-care; it's about carving out a space for yourself in this busy, beautiful new life.

Consider adding something to your humming ritual that feels special: a favorite spot to sit, a cozy blanket, or even lighting a candle. As you hum, let each vibration remind you that you're healing, that you're whole, and that you've brought something extraordinary into the world.

Keeping Humming in Your Self-Care Toolkit

You might wonder, "How long should I keep doing this?" And here's the thing—humming can be part of your life long after the postpartum haze has lifted. You've learned to use it as a calming tool, as a way to connect to yourself and your body. There's no expiration date on that.

As your baby grows, you'll find new moments to hum, to center yourself, to breathe. This technique is as much yours as it is theirs. And if someday you find yourself humming absentmindedly as they toddle around, you'll know you've created something special, a lasting connection that started with the gentle vibrations of sound.

Hummingbirth

Beyond Healing – Humming as Your Quiet Power

Humming isn't just about getting through labor or the first weeks of postpartum. It's about knowing you've got a simple, powerful tool that's always there when you need it. It's like carrying a little piece of wisdom with you, something ancient, yet perfectly suited to modern life.

As you hum through sleepless nights, through first smiles, through every milestone, know this: you've tapped into something timeless. You've found a way to harness calm, to carry yourself with a sound that's both strength and softness.

And that, dear reader, is the real magic of humming—it's not just a technique. It's part of you now. It's your own quiet power, a sound that can carry you through whatever comes next, one hum at a time.

Conclusion

And here we are, at the end of this little adventure together—except it's not an end, is it? You're still humming, your body still remembers, and those soft, gentle vibrations still have a role to play in your life, whether you're moments away from meeting your baby, wrangling toddlers, or years down the road. Because here's the thing: the hum is yours now.

If you take anything from this book—other than a sense of relief that labor doesn't have to be as scary as they make it out to be—I hope it's this: you are powerful beyond measure, even when you feel anything but. That power, that ancient knowledge buried deep in your cells, has always been there. Humming just gives you a way to access it, to bring it out into the open.

The Hum as Revolution

Here's something wild to consider: you're part of a long line of women who've labored, birthed, nurtured, and hummed before you, all drawing on that same quiet strength. In your most tender, tired moments, remember that you're connected to something big, something almost primal. To hum is to tap into a source of calm that's as old as time. It's practically revolutionary in a world that tells us to do more, be more, go faster.

Imagine this: you, sitting there humming, practicing calm, choosing a slower, kinder way to bring life into the world. Choosing connection over chaos, gentleness over fear. That hum isn't just a sound; it's a declaration. You're telling the world you trust your body, you trust birth, and you trust the wisdom that comes from within.

Life, in All Its Messy, Humming Glory

Of course, life isn't always calm and collected. It's sticky floors, unwashed hair, and endless "why" questions from small humans who can't find their shoes but can locate a candy wrapper from 2017 in under three seconds. And that's why I love the hum. It's the anti-perfection, the low-key, low-maintenance trick for keeping it together.

Because here's the honest truth: you won't always feel strong. You won't always feel like the warrior mama or the serene goddess. Some days, you'll feel like a tired human who just wants five minutes of quiet. But in those moments, remember the hum. Because if there's anything I've learned, it's that the hum is your tether.

The Simple Sound of Grace

There's a certain grace in humming, a quiet surrender to whatever is happening in that moment. The hum isn't loud; it doesn't shout. It's a small, steady thing, vibrating just beneath the surface. It's a reminder that sometimes strength doesn't have to look like boldness. Sometimes, it's just showing up, breathing deep, and making the choice to hum through whatever life brings your way.

As you move forward, know this: you have the power to hum through it all. Whether you're facing a contraction or a sleepless night, a job change, or a Tuesday that just won't quit. The hum is with you, a reminder that you are capable, that you can find peace, that you are enough.

So, as you close this book, maybe you'll take a second to hum, to let that sound fill your chest, soften your shoulders, settle into your bones. Know that with each hum, you're creating a rhythm

Hummingbirth

of calm, a song that's just for you—a song of resilience, grace,
and strength that will carry you forward, one hum at a time.

Congratulations, dear reader. You've got this. The hum is yours,
and with it, you're ready for whatever comes next.

References

(1) L.J. Seltzer, T. E. Ziegler, and S.D. Pollack. "Social Vocalization Can Release Oxytocin Humans," *Proceedings of the Royal Society B; Biological Sciences 277, No 1694 (2010): 2661-66*

(2) Health Essentials; *health.clevelandclinic.org, March 10th, 2022*

(3) Eddie Weitzberg and John O. N. Lundberg, "Humming Greatly Increases Nasal Nitric Oxide", *American Journal of Respiratory and Critical Care Medicine 166, no. 2 (2002): 144-45*

(4) *Seltzer, Ziegler, and Pollak, "Social Vocalizations Can Release Oxytocin in Humans."*

(5) *K. Pederson,' Bhramari Pranayama (Humming Bee Breath)," December 17, 2012, http://www.yogawiz.com/articles/83/yoga-breathing-pranayama/bhramari.html*

(6) *T. Pramanik, B. Pudasaini, and R. Prajapati, Nepal Medical College Journal 12, no. 3 (September 2110): 154-57*

Recommended Resources

To my knowledge, *Hummingbirth* is the first in-depth book ever written about the profound connection between humming and childbirth. Because of this, I can't recommend any other books specifically on this subject—yet! However, there is one book that deeply influenced my journey and laid the foundational inspiration to birth the Hummingbirth Method: *The Humming Effect* by Jonathan and Andi Goldman.

This remarkable book opened my eyes to the transformative power of humming—not just as a sound, but as a tool for healing, connection, and profound personal transformation. It planted the seed that grew into the Hummingbirth Method and, ultimately, the creation of this book. Reading *The Humming Effect,* combined with my decades of experience in sound therapy, healing, and midwifery, reignited my passion and gave me a renewed sense of purpose. It inspired me to reimagine childbirth as an opportunity for empowerment, connection, and profound change, both for mothers and their children.

I cannot recommend *The Humming Effect* enough for anyone curious about the science and soul behind humming. This book is a treasure, and I am deeply grateful for the spark it gave me. It is my hope that *Hummingbirth* continues that spark in your own journey, helping you approach childbirth—and life itself—with a new sense of calm, strength, and possibility. Together, these books offer a powerful path back to our roots, reminding us of the beauty and wisdom already within us.

It feels only fitting to conclude this page with an excerpt from *The Humming Effect*. After all, there is no prayer more profound, no sacred song more powerful, than the sound of a mother calling her baby earthside.

Hummingbirth

"There is a reason why almost all prayers on this planet are vocalized---whispered, chanted, read aloud, spoken, or sung. It is this: Sound amplifies the power of prayer. Prayer amplifies the power of sound. Together, sound and prayer (intention, thought, belief) build a mutually reinforcing feedback loop. It is that simple and that important."

Download your Complimentary Guided Hummingbirth Meditation Here:
www.hummingbirththemethod.com

www.ingramcontent.com/pod-product-compliance
Lightning Source LLC
Chambersburg PA
CBHW050829250726
48653CB00006B/2503